Becoming "Mom": My Fight Against Infertility
By Bianca Clovis

Chapter 1

I was eleven when I got my period. I was at the mall when it happened. I had just finished lunch in the food court and I had gone into the bathroom. When I pulled down my underwear there was a spot of blood the size of a quarter.

I had older friends so I knew what a period was. I was glad mine had come so early. It made me feel grown up.

The only bad thing about getting my period was that my mom was on a trip for work and I didn't have anyone to show me how to use a sanitary pad. At least, that was what I thought was the worst of it at the time.

Ten days later I was still bleeding. Not quarter sized droplets but blood that flowed over the edges of my pad and soiled my clothes.

My mom, who was finally home from her trip, called the doctor.

"It's common for girls to have irregular periods at first," Dr. Z told my mom. "Have her keep track of the days she bleeds and if the flow is heavy or light. In a few cycles we will probably see them normalizing."

Eleven was the bloodiest year of my life. I would bleed for four or five weeks. Then, I would have a five day respite before the bleeding began again. After a year it still hadn't normalized as my doctor had hoped.

"We will put her on birth control pills for a few years. It will teach her body what it is supposed to do," Dr. Z said.

At twelve years old I started taking a little white pill every night before bed so that my body could see how periods were supposed to be. I didn't really think much about it at the time. I believed my doctor knew what to do and that it must have been a common problem. I was sure the pills would fix it. Once I was off of the birth control pills my periods would be like everyone else's. I would bleed for a week like my friends. I would then not have to worry about my period for another month.

Of course, that was just the beginning. The first hint that my reproductive system was flawed.

I remained on birth control pills until I got married.

I married my high school sweetheart. We were both eighteen at the time.

I had met Slim at school my junior year. He was a senior. He was tall and rail thin. He liked to dress in all black at school and listen to heavy metal. We had lunch period and study hall together. He was a friend of a friend. I was sixteen when we met and for the first time ever I was glad I was on birth control pills already. We didn't have to fumble around with condoms nor did I have to admit to my mom that I had decided I was ready to start having sex and needed the pills as a contraceptive.

I had a husband, my own apartment, and a dog. The next logical step was a baby. I had two friends who had accidentally gotten pregnant while in high school. I often hung out with them and their babies. Being around them made me want to have a cute little baby of my own.

Slim wasn't as keen on starting a family so soon but he was a very 'go with the flow' type of guy. So, when I stopped taking my birth control he just went with it.

I had two normal periods and I thought my six years on birth control must indeed have fixed the problems I had experienced. Then, my period didn't come. I was elated. I went out and bought a pregnancy test. Excitedly, I followed the directions and peed on the little wand and waited. Negative? How could it be negative? I was a week late on my period. Another week passed. Then another. Then a month. Still, no period. Then, it came. With a vengeance. After six weeks of bleeding I picked up a packet of birth control pills and took the first white pill.

Why was my body still confused?

I scheduled an appointment with a gynecologist. I had seen one for a routine pap smear before we were married but he had been on my parents insurance plan. I had gotten my own insurance and so had to choose a new doctor.

At Dr. W's I filled out a ton of paperwork. He glanced over it and ordered an ultrasound. He did a pelvic exam as well.

"I don't see anything wrong. Just keep trying to get pregnant. Pregnancy will straighten things out," he said. I could barely understand his words through his heavy accent.

I stopped taking the birth control pills again. And again, I had two normal cycles. The next two months I had no periods and negative pregnancy tests. Then, the torrential bleeding started again.

'Maybe I can ride it out,' I thought. Maybe, we can keep trying once the bleeding stops. If my period reverted to four weeks of bleeding and a weeks respite Slim and I could still try during that single week.

After bleeding for nine weeks straight I couldn't take it any more. I picked up the birth control again. I was in tears as I popped the white pill into my mouth.

For the next year and a half I would take my birth control for two months. Then, I would stop taking it and we would try to conceive during the two or rarely even three months where I had normal cycles.

Emotionally, it was tearing me up inside. More of my friends were getting pregnant as we entered our twenties. Slim and I had bought a house with two bedrooms. I had already planned out the nursery in my head. We were using the room as a computer room but I wouldn't let Slim clutter up the room. After all, we were trying. Any month I could be late and have a positive pregnancy test and we would need to clear out the computer desk and replace it with a crib and changing table.

I decided I needed a second opinion. I didn't want to go back to Dr. W. I thought maybe the language barrier had created some miscommunication that could explain why we still weren't getting pregnant.

I made an appointment to see Dr. L after being assured that English was his first language. I signed a release of information so he could get copies of my ultrasound from Dr. W and I filled out the required paperwork.

Dr. L sauntered into the room with my chart in hand. He was a youngish man. Probably in his thirties. He didn't order any tests nor did he give me any kind of exam. With a single glance he had his "diagnosis".

"You are overweight. You need to lose weight. That's why you can't get pregnant."

"But, my periods have always been irregular," I said.

"Have you always been overweight?" he asked. I nodded. I had been a chunky child. I had grown into a chunky teenager and an obese adult. According to his charts I was about 100 lbs over my ideal weight.

"Lose the weight and you will get pregnant."

"I'm willing to do that," I said. "But isn't there anything we can do in the meantime."

"I will not treat you until you lose weight. I'm not saying that you don't have other problems but I won't do anything for you to help you get pregnant at your current weight."

I had other friends who were my weight and had gotten pregnant with no problems. But, I didn't argue.

I started taking my birth control again. I started to exercise and I joined Weight Watchers. It took me a year to lose 50 lbs. We had moved by then because of Slim's job and I went to a new gynecologist to establish care. Dr. H was the first female gynecologist I had ever seen. I told her my history and explained that I was trying to lose weight so I could get pregnant.

"Have you ever been on Metformin?" she asked.

"No," I said.

"It is a medicine for patients with diabetes but one of the side effects they found during testing was that some women who were previously infertile became pregnant."

"I'm not diabetic," I said.

"Putting you on Metformin won't hurt you and it might help you."

After a 50 lb weight loss and two months on Metformin I again stopped my birth control. When my period was late on the third month I didn't even bother to take a pregnancy test. They were too expensive and getting a negative result hurt too much. Instead, I waited. Sure enough, my period came and decided to stay. Discouraged, I picked up my birth control and popped the first pill of the packet.

Even with weight loss and Metformin I still had to be on birth control in order to not bleed all the time. Obviously, I wasn't going to get pregnant while taking birth control. That went against the whole point of birth control.

I called my doctor. She said we could meet in a few months and talk about other options. But, before our appointment could happen, Slim and I realized that we needed to get a divorce.

Slim and I loved each other. But, we had grown into very different people. He and I didn't want the same things in life. We were no longer able to live harmoniously together. So, heavy hearted, we ended our marriage. I can honestly say that Slim and I had the friendliest divorce I had ever heard of. We didn't fight over anything during the divorce and we remained best friends after.

Chapter 2

I was in my mid twenties, single, and still desperate to be a mom. I started looking into my options. Fertility treatments with artificial insemination was way out of my price range. Besides, I come from a very conservative and religious family and purposefully being single and pregnant would have given my parents a heart attack.

I was pretty sure I didn't want a husband again. I had dated a little since Slim and I had separated but the men I had met in my age group were not the men I wanted to build a life with. Most were immature and wanted to spend their evenings drinking and smoking pot instead of changing diapers and balancing a check book. I had decided that I was going to have to be a parent alone. And, I was okay with that decision.

Since artificial insemination wasn't an option and neither was marriage I started looking into adoption.

This road had almost as many roadblocks as finding a husband and artificial insemination had. Private adoptions could get you a baby in theory. But, most single women giving up a newborn would not want to place their baby with a single woman working a dead end job. At the time I worked in the hospitality industry. I knew that if I had been a young woman placing a baby for adoption I would have wanted a married couple where the mother would be able to stay home with the baby.

International adoption would have eliminated the issue of my being a single woman. In most international adoption situations the biological parents are not consulted about the placement of their child. It wouldn't matter that I was a single woman. I was a woman willing to take a child from a crowded orphanage. But, the price for an international adoption made it impossible for me. I talked to several agencies and the price for the adoption would have been equal to my yearly gross pay. Also, each country has their own policies about who could adopt a child. For instance, when I was looking into adoption I was told that China would not allow people with a BMI (Body Mass Index) over a certain number. I was still obese and my BMI was higher than they allowed.

The final adoption option was the one I decided I would take. Foster care adoption was financially feasible. But, it would mean I wasn't likely to have a newborn child. And, any child I adopted would have special needs whether physical or emotional.

Still, that seemed like the only path to motherhood for me. I started reading up on Fetal Alcohol Syndrome and Reactive Attachment disorder (two common problems with children adopted from the foster care system). I also started researching different physical and mental handicaps to see what I thought I could handle as a single woman.

Then, I went to family services to fill out an application to be put on their waiting families list.

I was denied.

Not enough time had passed since my divorce became official. I had to wait another ten months before I would be eligible to adopt.

I was sad but ten months wasn't forever. And, I had already waited more than 5 years for the child I wanted. What was another year?

I went back to college to get my associates degree so I could have better job opportunities. I also moved from my one bedroom apartment into a two bedroom townhouse and I started planning the room my son or daughter would stay in. I had decided to adopt a child around 5 years old. That way, they could be in school while I was at work. Daycare wouldn't be an issue. I had even put on my application that I would consider a sibling set. A seven year old and a five year old seemed doable. I knew I eventually wanted to have several children. These phantom children were always in my thoughts. They occupied my days as I got through school and long hours at work. When I was trying to get pregnant with Slim I had always fantasized about holding my newborn or playing with my toddler. As adoption became my expected path to parenthood my fantasies were of helping a five year old boy with his homework and watching his little league games.

But, in the months of waiting to be put on the adoption waiting list, something changed.

I met Junior.

Chapter 3

In my mid twenties I went back to the church I had been raised in. It was good to be back but it also made me desperate to turn my life around in a way that was pleasing to God.

Since my separation I had been intimate with a few men, including Slim. Slim was still my best friend and when he and I were both single we often hung out. Sometimes, the hanging out led to physical intimacy.

I like sex. I knew that quitting wasn't a viable option for me. But, I had the choice between abstinence, marriage, or sin. None of them good options.

Then, I met Junior. We met on a social networking website . He was the same religion I was which is how we started talking.

Junior was a handsome man but not what I normally went for. While Slim had been a my height and rail thin Junior was a mountain of a man. He was well over six feet tall and built like a body builder. His Elvin features seemed out of place on his muscular frame. He was in the army and he had just gotten back from a deployment in Iraq. His best friend had died and Junior had a new appreciation for life and his own mortality. He wanted a wife and kids before it was too late. A family to love him. To remember him if he died.

He was scheduled to deploy to Afghanistan the next year.

Junior and I started talking about our faith. Both of us were fairly new to church life. I was returning to it after having been away for almost ten years. He was new to church. It gave us common ground.

We found out we had both been home schooled for a time during our primary education. We both wanted a college education. I was currently in college and he had plans to start evening classes once his next deployment was finished.

We both loved animals and dreamed of owning a bit of land and homesteading.

And, most importantly, we both wanted children. Lots of children. I told him about my infertility and explained that I would need medical treatment to get pregnant and even then there were no guarantees. Adoption might be my only option.

Junior was fine with that. The military had great healthcare that would pay for fertility treatments (at least some of them) and a service to help with adoptions as well if we needed to go that route.

It seemed like we were a perfect match. We arranged for him to visit me in Ohio. He was stationed in Alaska.

He had to cancel a month before the visit because of mandatory training. He told me he didn't think there would be a good time for him to come and see me in Ohio. As the training intensified to prepare for deployment leave was getting hard to come by.

He had a different solution. He asked me to move to Alaska immediately and marry him. On paper, we were a perfect couple. We had been talking for months. And, our church encouraged marriage and took the stance that any couple who was devoted to God could form a happy marriage. I prayed about it for days before giving him my answer. In the best and worst decision of my life, I finally agreed to marry him.

I quit my job, dropped out of college, and jumped on a plane to Alaska.

In the airport I looked around for a tall muscled man. He was actually a bit more handsome in person though unsure of himself. We were both very awkward at first. I thought maybe he was disappointed with my looks. I got into his car afraid that when we got back to his house he was going to tell me that he had changed his mind and ship me back to Ohio. Or worse, make me find my own way.

I reached out and put my hand on his thigh. It was the first time we had ever touched. And, he almost wrecked the car.

The ice was broken and by the time we got home I knew that he and I were going to be husband and wife. We married six days later.

The wedding was small. It was performed by an army chaplain with just two witnesses in attendance. The witnesses were an army couple who also happened to attend church with Junior.

Chapter 4

I immediately stopped taking my birth control. Unfortunately, Junior wasn't very interested in sexual relations. But, I was sure he was just preoccupied with the upcoming deployment. Still, I got fairly frustrated that he wasn't able to put the effort into baby making that I thought we should be putting. I was married now. Married to a man who loved God. I had my life back on track. I was married and no longer fornicating. I thought maybe God hadn't given Slim and I a baby because He knew our marriage would fail. But, Junior and I were a solid couple. We were believers. Surely, God would bless us with a baby to raise in righteousness. I felt sure God would do that for us if we could just manage to have regular marital relations. But, sex kept not happening.

After six months of marriage, Junior went off to serve his country in Afghanistan. I was alone. In Alaska. I had no friends, nearby relatives, or job. The poor weather conditions and unfamiliarity with the area made me afraid to leave my home much of the time.

I suffered from depression and gained back the weight I had lost plus some.

Deployments are hard on the best marriages. It was extra hard on us. I was used to being married to my best friend. Slim and I had always communicated well. Even when we were no longer married I still knew what was happening in his life.

Communication with Junior all but stopped during the deployment. This was not due to lack of ability to communicate. I was in frequent contact with another army wife whose husband was stationed with mine. She was kind enough to inform me when my husband had pneumonia and couldn't work for a week. Her husband called her almost daily. Mine managed a five minute phone call every month.

Junior used the lack of communication to compartmentalize his situation. He was in Afghanistan. Anything back home would be nothing more than a distraction. I understood it but that didn't make it any easier for me to deal with.

The only consolation I had was that we would be moving

shortly after he came home. We would be going to Georgia which was only eleven hours away from my hometown. I would be close to my family again. I just had to make it through the deployment. Then, when he got home, we would have the life we dreamed of and the babies I desperately wanted.

Junior was sent home early from deployment due to an injury and put in the Wounded Warrior Program. As he recovered we were told he wasn't likely to deploy again in the near future. We decided it was as good a time as any to start trying for a baby.

I made an appointment to see an OBGYN and instead was handed over to a midwife.

Let me say that, overall, I think midwife's are wonderful. I have heard many good stories about the compassion of midwives. I was thrilled to see one.

"I can't do anything for you. You need to lose weight," she said.

This time, I was armed with research. I filed a complaint against the midwife and was put into the care of an OBGYN.

The OBGYN said that I should lose weight. But, there were other things to be done as well.

She performed a hysterosapingogram to check for blockage of my fallopian tubes. She found none. She started me on Chlomid.

Chlomid made me an emotional wreck. But, I found comfort in the fact that we were finally doing something. Something that would give me the child my heart had desired for so long..

I also asked to receive a healing blessing by a religious leader who was allowed to do such things at our church.

I was finally armed with a doctor who was doing something; a drug that would allow me to ovulate; and a bit of divine intervention. I was sure I would get pregnant.

We made it through the first cycle of Chlomid. On the days we were to have intercourse Junior and I were sick with colds. I was bummed to waste a whole cycle especially after the Chlomid had made me such an emotional wreck. I was sure we would have better luck the next month.

I went to have blood work and found that my body had not responded to the Chlomid. We would need to try a higher dose.

Before I started the next cycle of pills, Junior was in a serious car accident.

He came out of it with minor injuries but the other car had a fatality.

Bogged down in legal issues from the car accident and preparing for a move Junior sent me back to Ohio to stay with my family.

Chapter 5

Being home brought about it's own hardships. I was frustrated with Junior's lack of communication. I was concerned about our move and fearful of living in a city as big as the one we would be in.

To make the situation even more emotionally confusing, I saw Slim.

He and I had dinner the week of our wedding anniversary. He brought pictures of his niece and updated me on all the family news. One of his cousins had died in a tragic accident leaving her newborn an orphan to be raised by her aged parents.

Slim's parents had just separated and were preparing for divorce.

It was so nice to be communicating. To have the deep friendship. To feel close to Slim. We ended the night with a hug and we went our separate ways.

But, the seed of discontent was flowering within me.

Junior was the key to my future. He was the man who I was going to make babies with and be married to until death. Only, Junior couldn't even be bothered to call once a week. Packing the house for the move kept him too busy. Or so he claimed.

I sought out a faith based counselor and started seeing her. I told her my confusion. I had expected my marriage to Junior to have the same closeness as my marriage to Slim. Junior and I seemed so perfect on paper. Slim and I were so wrong on paper. Junior could give me the family I wanted. Slim had decided he didn't want to ever marry again. Nor did he want children. But, I wanted the closeness I only shared with Slim. The distance between Junior and I was growing by the day.

The counselor advised me not to give up on my marriage. Once we were settled Junior and I could attend couples counseling. We had just managed a deployment, a car accident, and a cross country move. That would be trying for any couple. Especially a couple who hadn't dated long before their marriage and hadn't had the time during the early part of their marriage to build normal couple bonds.

I was still devoted to God and to my marriage. I decided that Junior and I would work things out. And, as soon as we got to

Georgia we would start trying to start our family. I was sure that if I had Junior's baby I would be able to be content in our marriage. And, if I had a baby, it would mean that Slim and I had no hope of ever being together again. A baby would cut the ties that held my heart to his. I was sure of that. He didn't want children. He never dated women with children. Surely, once I was pregnant he and I would not even maintain a distant friendship. My life would be wound up in my baby and that would break us apart once and for all. And, it would cement Junior and I together. I was sure God was testing me. I just had to pass this one test. Get over this one speed bump. I just had to go to Georgia with my husband. As soon as possible I had to get my husband's child in my womb. If I did that, Slim would no longer be a temptation.

I found Junior and I a nice two bedroom apartment off post in Georgia. A perfect apartment for us to start our family in.

I immediately scheduled an appointment with my new primary care doctor. Before the appointment I wrote out a full history of my fertility struggles. I had also spent some time talking to other women who had struggled with infertility. I was prepared for the appointment.

The primary care doctor I had been assigned wasn't able to see me on my first visit. I would have to see her colleague instead. And, I truly believe that was an act of God.

I arrived at the appointment and gave her my written history. I was mentally armed and ready to battle.

"I'm going to refer you to Dr. V the fertility specialist. He is very good. He helped me to get pregnant when I was having trouble," she said. It was a miracle to me.

"Be sure you make an appointment immediately. They have a waiting list."

She was right. The next appointment I could get was three months away.

That was perfect, I thought. Enough time for Junior and I to get settled in our new home and to get counseling.

Chapter 6

I went alone on my first visit to Dr. V.

Dr. V was comparatively young. I guessed in his thirties. He was gorgeous. I totally had a crush on him from the first visit.

Dr. V was very professional and he put me at ease. He was foreign and spoke in accented English but his English was very good and I didn't have much trouble understanding him. In the rare instances I did he was happy to repeat himself.

I gave him my complete history including how I had some signs of polycystic ovarian syndrome (PCOS) but how my first doctor hadn't found evidence of it on an ultrasound.

It happened that Dr. V specialized in PCOS. He did an ultrasound and within fifteen minutes I had a diagnosis. I had PCOS. It was a fairly mild case. But, I had it for certain.

He explained to me that PCOS causes hormonal imbalances. I didn't have enough of some hormones and I had too much of others. The imbalances made ovulation irregular.

Obesity and PCOS go hand in hand and they feed each other. Women with PCOS find it very difficult to lose weight due to their imbalanced hormones. The obesity in turn makes the hormonal imbalances even worse.

Dr. V encouraged me to eat healthy and exercise. It was important for me to be as healthy as I could. But, my obesity wouldn't prevent him from treating me.

He needed Junior to contribute a sperm sample. Then, we could determine the best course of treatment.

"So, you will be able to help me?" I asked.

"Oh yes. I don't see any reason why you won't be able to have a baby."

Those words were the most beautiful I had ever heard.

I brought the good news back to Junior. I had scheduled another appointment with Dr. V to include Junior the next week. I had made it for a weekend so Junior wouldn't have trouble being there.

In the time since we had moved to Georgia to our first appointment with Dr. V Junior and I had made little progress in improving our marriage.

His new unit was preparing for a deployment to Afghanistan. We had already decided that I would return to Ohio to finish college while he was deployed.

I had explained to Dr. V that we had a time frame of only four months in which to try to conceive a baby. If we were not successful Junior would need to store his sperm in case he didn't make it through the next deployment. After the deployment we would try again.

The best choice would probably have been to have him store his sperm and wait until after the deployment to start trying. The problem was that I believed our marriage wouldn't survive another deployment like the last. Not unless I had a strong reason to stay with Junior. A baby would be the thread that held Junior and I together over another year without contact. By the time the deployment was over Junior and I would have been married for a little over 3 years. We would have spent two of those three years apart and with little communication.

Junior's new unit was much more demanding than his old one. He left for work before I woke up and he usually wasn't back until after six pm.

His weekends were spent hanging out with his fellow soldiers. He preferred I not meet his friends. Work life was work life and home life was home life.

When Junior was home all work topics were off limits. Including his work friends. The only thing we seemed to be able to talk about was the future we were trying to make together. It was the glue that bound us.

We had seen a marriage counselor for a few sessions but had ended up having to stop due to the cost. And I didn't feel that the counseling was helping. In the session I would explain my frustration with our lack of communication. I felt ignored. Unloved. I had heard about soldiers marrying to advance their careers and I sometimes was afraid that Junior had done that. I felt that marriage should mean emotional and physical intimacies. Junior assured me he had married me out of love. He vowed to make more time for me and to increase the intimacy in our marriage. But, no matter what he vowed during our sessions I never felt as if he followed through. I also didn't know what I could do to improve our marriage. I asked but he said he was very happy with the way things were and excited about our future.

The day of our joint appointment Junior was sullen and cranky.

"What's wrong?" I asked.

"Why do I have to get checked?" Junior asked.

"It's standard procedure," I explained. "If your sperm count is low or your swimmers are slow then the treatment will have to be adjusted."

"I really don't want to be tested."

"Why?" I asked. I had already had a series of painful and invasive tests. He only needed to ejaculate in a cup.

"You can't understand because you're a girl."

"Try to explain it?" I begged.

"It's like you are questioning my manhood," Junior said.

I have to admit that his comment infuriated me. It was all well and fine for me to be on my back on an exam table with hands and machines inside of me. He didn't know nor care about the shame I felt. My body didn't work. Without assistance I couldn't make a baby. Drunk fourteen year olds could make a baby. Heroine addicts could make a baby. A woman who had a one night stand at a bar could make a baby. My body couldn't. Not without help. But, Junior didn't want to have his boys evaluated because it was an insult to his penis?

"Do you want to have a baby?" I asked.

"Of course I do. But, we already know what the problem is. Why can't they just treat you?"

"If you want to have a baby this is what you have to do. Are you saying you won't do this? Are you saying your ego is so great that we just won't be able to have a baby because you don't want your penis questioned?"

"I didn't say that," Junior said. He was getting angry now too but I didn't care. I wasn't going to be denied a child just because my husband was a big soldier man who didn't want his masculinity questioned.

"The doctor won't treat us if you don't get tested too," I reminded him.

He glared at me for a good five minutes before answering me.

"I'll do it," he said grudgingly.

A sensible woman who wasn't as desperate for a baby as I was might have seen this exchange for the omen it was. But, I had tunnel vision. I had wanted a baby for almost eight years. And, I had just four months to have one or I would have to wait another year. A year that my marriage probably wouldn't survive. Afterwards, I would be almost thirty and no closer to having the baby I had been desperately trying for since I was eighteen.

I admit selfishness on my part. I was desperate for a baby. Desperate to stay married.

To make the situation even worse I had begun to question my faith. I had always believed in God and I had no doubts about him. It was my specific religion I was questioning. The rules. The things they declared a sin. I supported on a personal level many things that my church condemned such as gay marriage.

I was desperate for something to take the choices out of my hand. If I left my faith my marriage would crumble. My faith and my desire for a family was all that was holding Junior and I together. The lack of communication in our marriage had put up walls between Junior and I that were nearly insurmountable.

Slim and I had been best friends. Our marriage might have been turbulent and we might have wanted different things but we were always connected. Always.

Junior and I were strangers living together in a house. Our common goals were the only thing holding us together. And, they were holding us by a thread.

"Your sperm count and motility are fine," Dr. V said when Junior and I met in his conference room a week later.

"I would say even a bit above average." This made Junior beam. It was only my body that didn't work. It was only me who was broken.

Dr. V laid out a treatment plan for us. I was going to start on Metformin again. I was also going to take Chlomid on certain days of my cycle. Every four days I would come in for an ultrasound to see if my eggs were maturing.

He explained that ideally there would be several eggs maturing but most likely only one or two would get big enough to ovulate. Even in a release of multiple ripe eggs conception might not occur. The statistics were something like one in four times when an egg and sperm meet conception occurs. Not great odds.

I started the Metformin. It gave me nausea, diarrhea, and stomach cramps. The Chlomid put me on an emotional roller coaster.

As Dr. V kept checking me it became apparent that I wasn't responding to the treatment.

"We need to up the dosage," he said. We did. More medicine equaled stronger side effects. I was an emotional wreck and we hadn't even completed a full cycle.

With the increased Chlomid I responded. A little. I had an egg. A single egg that seemed to be growing adequately.

I started taking urine ovulation tests. If the test was positive Junior and I would need to hop into bed and attempt to make a baby. But, the test never was positive. At the next visit to Dr. V he took blood samples to see if my hormones were where they needed to be to ovulate. They weren't. I would need an injection to force the ovulation.

"I think we are going to need to be more aggressive," Dr. V explained. If you don't get pregnant this cycle I think we need to start injections. You will give yourself the injections into your abdomen. Then, once the egg or eggs are large enough we will need to use an injection in your gluteus maximus to force ovulation."

The nurse showed Junior how to give the injection into my rear. Being a soldier, injections weren't new to him.

The doctor told us which days we would need to engage in intercourse and we left the office.

The prescribed days came and Junior was too tired. His work days had been too long. He just couldn't manage the act.

"Are you sure you want to keep trying? Are you not ready for a baby?" I asked him as we laid in bed and he had removed my offending hand from his flaccid penis.

"I do want a baby. I just had a rough week at work. And I keep remembering stuff that happened in Afghanistan. I was sexually assaulted," he said. He was facing the wall when he said it. I didn't know what the correct answer to that was.

"Oh," I said. "Do you want to talk about it?"

"No," he said gruffly. Then he went to sleep.

Chapter 7

My period came and went and I started the injections.

During this time my niece had a birthday party. She was turning two. My sister lived about six hours from us in Kentucky. Junior couldn't get leave to go to the party so I went by myself. I arrived the day before to help my sister set up.

My sister was going through a divorce and I was worried about Junior and my marriage. How had he not told me about being assaulted? What kind of assault was it?

Plus, I had noticed missing money in our checking account and knew Junior had been lying about where is had gone.

My sister and I decided we both needed a drink.

After my niece was safely in bed I went out to purchase a few "bitch drinks." Fruity flavored drinks that would knock us on our asses. I brought the bottles home and my sis and I started taste testing them.

Neither my sister or I drank much. The religion we had been raised in forbade alcohol consumption. During my non religious days I had had an occasional drink with a friend but I had never gotten drunk. But, that night, I wanted to.

It didn't take long for me to feel dizzy and nauseated. I hadn't thought about the effects of alcohol with the metformin and fertility medicines. I still had at least another week before ovulation so I wasn't worried about the effects of the alcohol on a child. It would be out of my system by the next day.

As the effects of the alcohol made me sick and giddy I decided to text Slim. Since our divorce he had partied some. Less then once a month at his peek time. But, he would understand. Junior hated alcohol and would be appalled at my consumption.

Not to mention the fact that I was sinning by consuming the alcohol. I was a Sunday school teacher he would have reminded me. Sunday school teachers didn't get drunk. Not even with their sisters who needed it.

I didn't throw up and by the next afternoon when my parents arrived for the party there was no evidence of our "fun" the night before.

But, two things kept niggling at my conscience.

The first was that I had drank which was a sin. But, I wasn't feeling particularly guilt ridden over it.

The second was that I had wanted to talk to Slim when I was drunk. He would understand me. Junior wouldn't. It didn't seem like Junior and I were understanding each other much at that point.

I finally had the life I had always thought I wanted.

I was a married woman. I was a homemaker. I was on my way to having a baby. I was an active member of my church.

But, I was miserable. Junior and I weren't getting along and I hated my life.

Maybe it was all the hormones, I thought. Maybe it was the stress of trying to conceive. Or, maybe it was my sense that my marriage to Junior was doomed.

In two months I would be moving back to Ohio to finish school. Junior had just gotten word that he wouldn't be deploying due to his health issues just a few days before. But, I was still going to finish college. In three classes I would have an associate's degree.

I kept telling myself that distance would help Junior and I communicate better. We would spend evenings on the phone like we had when we dated. I wouldn't feel ignored when he came home, played his video games, and then went to bed. Also, our lack of a sexual relationship wouldn't be an issue. Especially with trying to conceive it was a huge point of contention between us. I didn't know if he was having an affair, gay, not into sex, or just not into me.

And, I would finally have things to talk about. In Ohio I would be working and in school. The fact that he refused to talk about his work day wouldn't eliminate all chances of conversation between us. I would be able to carry the conversation.

It was true that Slim would be only an hour away from where I was living and that caused a slight twinge of worry in the sensible part of my soul. But, as a whole, it brought relief. I would be an hour away from my best friend. He wouldn't ignore me. We could go out together. He wouldn't have soldiers to worry about that would prevent us from spending an evening at the arcade or any other activities that Junior never had time for.

Chapter 8

"You are still not responding to the treatment. We are really going to need to increase your dosage next cycle. I see one mature egg. There are two small ones but I doubt they will grow enough to ovulate in the next few days. Tomorrow, do the injection. Then, you will need to have sex Monday and Wednesday. Here is a prescription for progesterone suppositories. You will need to insert one of these into your vagina each night before going to bed. With PCOS it is common for progesterone levels to be too low to sustain early pregnancy," Dr. V said.

It just isn't meant to be I thought. My marriage isn't strong enough. God knows how things are between Junior and I. He knows we aren't going to make it. He is just trying to keep me from having a baby from a broken family.

We left without filling the progesterone prescription. I only had one egg after all. I wasn't responding to the medicine.

The next night Junior gave me the injection. It was the first time he had given me one and I was sure he had done it wrong because it hurt. It hadn't really hurt when the nurse had done the injection the month before but this injection made me cry.

Monday night came.

"We need to do this," I said.

"Baby, I had a rough day at work," Junior said. That was it. The hormones and my own frustration came to the surface.

"You will do this Junior. I don't care how tired you are. I don't care how rough your day was. You will do this or so help me God I will go to the nearest bar and find someone who will." I don't think I had ever been so cruel or savage with Junior. As a rule, I didn't argue with him. It didn't have any effect other than to upset me anyways. My marriage to Slim had been full of heated arguments and shouting matches. Junior and I just didn't communicate. We didn't meet each others needs.

Without foreplay or joy Junior did what needed done. We were both relieved when he ejaculated and it was all over.

In a temper I turned over to sleep. Then, a thought started niggling at me.

"Did you not want to because of what happened in Afghanistan," I asked softly. Putting a hand against his back in a gesture of comfort.

"What are you talking about?" he asked.

"You said you had been sexually assaulted in Afghanistan," I said gently.

"No I didn't," Junior said. "That didn't happen."

"You did say that," I insisted.

"I think you dreamed that," he said with annoyance. I rolled over to let him sleep.

I knew I hadn't dreamed it. It was just another lie Junior had told. Although, I didn't know what was true. Had it been true when he told me he was assaulted or when he said he wasn't. Did he even know which lies were the truth. He had suffered a head injury overseas. I conceded that maybe his memory had been effected.

Something was wrong. Otherwise, why were there so many lies that Junior was tangled in.

Tuesday, Junior decided we should go out to dinner. Thursday I would be leaving in the morning for Ohio to find an apartment to stay in while I went to school.

"I don't think the army will let me reenlist. They are worried about my health," Junior said.

"How do you feel about that?" I asked. Junior loved being a soldier.

"I'm fine with it. I want to go to school. There is something I didn't tell you about when I was unconscious and they were flying me from Afghanistan to Germany."

"Oh?" I asked. I wanted to be interested but I also wasn't sure I wanted to hear what Junior had to say. Maybe because of the intensity in his voice. The plea for me to understand.

"I had a vision. A Heavenly Messenger came to me. He showed me this thing. I'm supposed to build it. It will make the US no longer dependant on foreign oil," Junior said.

"Wow," was the only response I could manage.

"That's why I need to go to school. People have tried to build this before and the government assassinated them. It is really dangerous. But, I will do everything I can to protect you and the kids."

"Thanks," I said. Now, I had a dilemma. I believed in God. I believed that the stories from the bible were true. I believed that God had spoken to man and still could. But, I didn't believe he had spoken to Junior. I didn't believe that Junior had been called to build any kind of scientific device. I didn't even know if Junior had really had a dream of some kind or if the vision was just another of his lies.

"Well, once I am done with school we can concentrate on your schooling," I said. Although, I didn't believe it.

Junior hadn't been honest with our councilors when we were seeking help. He hadn't been forthcoming with his doctors and when I had tried to get involved he had pushed me away. There was no way he would get treatment for whatever issues he was having. And, I wasn't strong enough to live with the constant lies. I knew that.

On Wednesday night when he refused to have sex I didn't press the issue. I wasn't meant to have a baby. Not with him. I was sure of it. Not after he had just admitted to having visions from God. We weren't going to make it. I was sure of that. I was going to finish school and then Junior and I could reevaluate our situation. Perhaps, the doctors would have found something by then and have some treatment options. More likely, I could simply walk away from the marriage after he didn't bother calling for three months.

Thursday, I went back to Ohio. My parents were out of town for the weekend so I stayed with Slim. We were up late that night as I told him the woes of my marriage and about the vision Junior had told me of. We almost slept together. He was lonely and so was I. But, I wouldn't without a condom because of the fertility treatments.

We hadn't had sex since I had started dating Junior. It had been almost four years. But, neither Slim nor I liked condoms and we decided that it wasn't a good idea. We had just been caught up in the moment I told myself.

We hung out Friday.

Then, Saturday, we went to his nieces' birthday party.

Something changed in me during the party. I had missed Slim. Missed his family. It felt right. It felt like being home to be there with them.

I still loved Slim. And I knew that Junior and me were never going to make it. No matter how hard we tried.

After we got home from the party Slim and I threw caution to the wind and we had sex. It was the best sex of my life. Years of missing each other and love all were built up. We were full of need and of love. I knew that no one would ever get me the way Slim did. I didn't know if Slim and I had a future. But, I knew Junior and I didn't.

Sunday, my parents came home and I spent a week visiting them and preparing to move home for school.

I was getting ready to go back to Georgia to say goodbye and pack my things. I would have a little over a month in Georgia.

Then, the day I was supposed to leave, I woke up violently sick. I was sick for almost a week. And that was when I realized that my period hadn't come.

I called Dr. V's office and said I wouldn't be up for my follow up appointment because I was ill. The nurse asked if my menstrual cycle had started and I told her that it hadn't but I had been very sick and knew that could make a period late.

"Not with the medicines you were on. You need to take a pregnancy test."

"I'm in Ohio and I can't drive right now," I said.

"Dr. V can send an order to your hospital for a blood draw."

I agreed grudgingly.

I couldn't be pregnant. Dr. V had said I wasn't responding to the treatment. There had only been one egg. And, Junior and I had only had sex once. Not on both of the appointed days. And, to top it all off I hadn't even used the progesterone suppositories because I was so sure I wasn't going to get pregnant.

I called Junior to tell him I was going to take a test. I also called one of my best girlfriends who had struggled with infertility. She knew how much I dreaded going in and paying for a pregnancy test just to have another negative. Every time that happened it broke my heart.

I went and did the test. Part of me was sure it would be negative. But, the part that wondered if it could be positive was in a panic.

I had just cheated on Junior. After his revelation about the vision I didn't think I could make the marriage work. And, I didn't want to. I was done. I knew I couldn't make any kind of life with Junior. Not one where I could thrive anyways. But, if there was a baby...

Dr. V's nurse called me to give me the news.

Even with my emotional turmoil my joy was so great that I shouted and jumped up and down.

I was going to be a mom. And, I instantly knew I was going to have a girl.

I called Junior and then I sent texts all of my friends, including Slim.

That message made me sad. I was going to be a mom. Slim didn't want children. Didn't like them. Wouldn't be with a woman with children. The last night we had been together was it. The last chapter for us. It broke my heart.

But, I knew Junior and I weren't going to make it either. I couldn't raise a daughter in a home with someone who took our money and was not willing to get help for his mental conditions. I was losing both the men I had loved but I was gaining a baby. My sweet, long awaited baby. My daughter.

Chapter 9

In Georgia I prepared my things for the move. I also went with Junior shopping for baby things. It was an awful experience.

He would look at the price tag of a necessary item and complain about what new thing he could get for his car at the same cost. He was trying to turn his little Honda Civic into a race car. I had been angry about his desire to have a race car when we were not financially stable but it had been just another argument we didn't have. Now, I hated the car. I hated that Junior was more concerned about the remodeling of his car then about having a stroller and a crib for his child.

I knew that my daughter would only have one person looking out for her interests. And that person was me. Even poor and single I would put my daughter first. I wouldn't let Junior spend her diaper money on things to improve his car.

In the morning before I left for Ohio for the last time, I had an ultrasound.

Dr. V had wanted to make sure that the pregnancy was in the uterus and to see if there was cardiac activity. Conception didn't automatically mean a baby and he was quick to remind me of that. I still could miscarry.

Junior was with me at the ultrasound and held my hand.

"Let me see her chart," Dr. V said to the nurse. He looked over his notes carefully and I could feel the panic rising. Was I not pregnant after all? Had the test been wrong.

"This isn't supposed to be like this," Dr. V said.

"What's wrong?" Junior asked. He could sense my concern and genuine concern was on his face as well.

"There are two. You are having two babies."

Dr. V turned the monitor to us and we could see two little heartbeats.

Uh oh I thought. I only had one egg that was ready to be ovulated on my last visit. Did one of the smaller ones finish growing later? Could it have dropped a few days after the first. Could one of my babies be Junior's and the other Slim's?

As soon as I was out in the car I sent a text to Slim and I

promised I would call my new gynecologist to ask if such a thing was even possible.

Her answer "If you had sex with both men within a ten day period then the babies could belong to either. And, it is possible for one baby to belong to each father."

Epilogue:

God is wonderful, merciful, and has a sense of humor.

Junior and I drifted apart during my pregnancy. Slim and I grew closer.

Junior proved to me time and again that he wasn't the man I wanted to raise my children with. He didn't even come up when the kids were born because he wanted to use the gas money to replace something on his car.

A DNA test after my twin daughter's birth showed that they both were the biological children of Junior. But, by then, Slim was in love.

I filed for divorce from Junior. He was given visitation rights he rarely uses.

When the girls were four months old Slim was having issues at work and I was having issues with daycare.

Slim quit his job and we moved in with him. He became a full time stay at home dad. And, he is amazing at it. As of this writing we have been in this arrangement for more than two years.

Slim and I have no plans to marry. I want another child but doing fertility treatments again is out of the question. I am currently trying to lose weight. Maybe, if I ever get to my ideal weight, God will give me another miracle.

My girls are thriving. They were born premature and have some developmental delays but I wouldn't trade them for anything.

And my faith in God remains but is changed.

I believe only God could have pulled off our situation.

If Slim and I hadn't slept together and if I hadn't had twins (which I wasn't supposed to and which made me worry that one of the kids could belong to Slim) then I would probably be a single mom.

If Slim wasn't having issues with his work I don't think we would have moved in together and my girls wouldn't have the awesome dad that they do.

Our family isn't perfect. But, in my eyes, it is a miracle from God.

On the other hand, I don't go to church anymore. I don't need to be reminded that I am a sinner. I did the best I could for my kids even if it meant sinning. I can't regret my actions. And, I can't regret the life I have now. My kids have a loving and involved father even though he isn't related to them by blood.

Slim and I are still best friends. He makes me happier than Junior ever could have.

My journey through infertility was a long and difficult one. But, I have two amazing daughters from it and I wouldn't do anything different.

Bianca's tips for overcoming infertility:

If you have any problems with your reproductive system consult a doctor. I wish my mom would have taken me to a doctor when I was 11. Maybe, I could have gotten a head start on heading off the issues I had.

Be educated. If what the doctor says doesn't sound right it probably isn't.

Be your own advocate. Know what you want and be willing to fight for it. No one cares about your fertility as much as you do.

Be in the best health YOU can be in before you try to conceive. Let me be clear here. I think if you are trying to conceive and you are overweight it is good to be exercising and changing your eating habits. I don't think you should wait until you are at your "ideal" weight before getting the help you need to conceive.

If you are having a baby with a partner make sure your relationship is solid before you start. Fertility treatment is tough. It is even tougher if you and your partner are at odds.

See a specialist if you think you need it. There are some amazing OBGYN doctors in the world. I know several people who have been able to conceive with the help of just an OBGYN. But sometimes more is needed. I wish that I had been sent to a specialist long before I was. It would have saved me so many years of heartache.

There are so many kinds of fertility treatments. If you can afford the treatments you can have a baby. In the absolute worst case scenario there is the option of donor sperm, donor egg, and a surrogate mother. If a baby is truly your hearts desire and you are willing to work for it then you will be a parent.

Consider adoption as an alternative. It was really helpful knowing that I was going to have a child one way or another. It took some of the pressure off of trying to conceive. I was friends with another couple who were having difficulties conceiving but they had decided that if a child wasn't of their DNA then they would just be childless. That is a personal choice and I don't condemn them for it but I can say there was less pressure on me then on them because I knew I would have my hearts desire even if every treatment failed.

Feel blessed even if things don't turn out quite as you had planned or hoped for. God has a plan. We just don't always understand what that plan is.

Seek counseling if you need it to deal with the emotional turmoil of infertility. It is hard to want a child and not be able to have one easily. It is horrible having negative pregnancy tests. It is painful to watch your friends grow up and have babies while you grow older and remain childless.

Be financially stable and have money saved up for fertility treatments. They are expensive.

Bianca Clovis can be emailed at biancaclovis@hotmail.com

Thanks for reading.

If you enjoyed this book please consider leaving a review on the retail website of your choice.

Other Books By Bianca Clovis:

Bianca's Guide to Twins: Pregnancy
11 Mistakes Couples Make During
Deployments

www.ingramcontent.com/pod-product-compliance
Lightning Source LLC
Chambersburg PA
CBHW030550290526
45786CB00004B/1950